Happy Labor Day

Katy Frank

Happy Labor Day

Katy Frank

ISBN 978-0-578-36509-1

Happy Labor Day: A BirthCare Story of Labor and Childbirth

Cover art by Joseph Patton

Contents

Dedication

To all the pregnant people everywhere on planet Earth

Childbirth is a marathon. It is hard work, and if you are like me you don't want to run a marathon every day. Or more than a few times. Or maybe ever. But when you cross this finish line you will feel a pride like none other ever before in your life. Plus, it will give you the perfect excuse to eat a whole box of doughnuts and drink a bottle of wine, or whatever refreshment makes you happy.

Gratitude

My first song of praise is to Priyanka Walunjkar, the artist who painted my body with mehndi, or henna, when I was eight months pregnant with my second child. Priyanka brought this beautiful, ancient ritual to my home and filled me with a sense of celebration and strength at a time when I needed to thrive during the raw and transcendent experience of childbirth. Henna is believed to keep the "evil eye" from the baby and child bearer, and is associated with positive spirits, prosperity and good luck.

Staining my body with mehndi at that time was also fortuitous because of its cooling properties and its meaning as a celebration of the sun, as my second child was born during a blazing hot summer and we had decided to name her Fiammetta, which means "small fire or flame."

I would be remiss if I did not turn next to thank all the family and friends and colleagues and even strangers who cleaned and cooked and performed other small miracles during my postpartum recoveries, most notably my husband Jacob, my mother Jill Rinaldi, my godmother Fran Pullano, Dee Dee McCabe, my brother Steven, my brother-in-law Joseph, Leita and Jerry Patton, and the magical lactation consultants from The Breastfeeding Center for Greater Washington.

Now I must extend arms of recognition to the generous women who assisted with these births and/or reviewed these stories:

Elin Shartar, CNM; Amy Patten, NP; Lori Cooper; Kerry Spinks; Theresa Noll; Dr. Sarah Minegar; Holly Poole-Kavana; Martha Weaver, CNM; Dorothy Lee, CNM; Marsha Jackson, CNM; Annie Rohlin, CNM; and Carrie Camillo

And finally, I bow with gratitude to BirthCare and Women's Health in Alexandria, Virginia for tending to me when I was pregnant, when I wasn't pregnant, and everything in between. You listened, advised, and empowered me— three things that always make all the difference in this experience of being human.

Our Oral Tradition

Allow me to begin by saying that I did not write this to dictate how you should give birth, or how to be a parent. We must all do our best with the body we have, and with the time and resources and luck at our disposal. And luck is not often a gentle lady. Sometimes her hormones go nuts, and she turns into a bully dragon and takes a big flying reptilian dump all over us. But we persevere and propagate the human race despite all the fire that is spat in our direction.

This is just my own reasonable, true story of pregnancy and childbirth. No more, no less. I call it reasonable because although I did not give birth in the midst of multiple orgasms while perched on a bed of lotus flowers, I can honestly say I had two wonderful births and I believe that you can, too.

That being said, I recognize that I was situated to enjoy many benefits during labor and childbirth — a group of midwives and birth assistants who not only respected my body as my own, but empowered me to make choices and helped me feel heard; babies who had the good sense to move, maintain a heartbeat and get their heads down so that labor could go smoothly; comprehensive medical insurance; and good physical health, which enabled me to give birth two times outside of a hospital. I know many child bearers face an uphill battle because one, several, or all of these benefits are not in place for them. I also believe we must take action wherever we can as a society to make that better.

I wrote this story because I prepared for childbirth by listening to my mother, my mother-in-law, my grandmother, and my aunts and cousins and friends who gave birth before me and were generous enough to tell me their tales. I wrote it because, although every child bearer's birth experience is unique, birth is a story that binds us together like an unbreakable vow. It binds us all the way back in time to the first hairy upright female homo sapiens. It binds us all the way around the planet to every childbearing person who shares the Earth with us today. As my own mom says, "Mothers know no strangers." Welcome to the mama ship.

When my friend Kerry gave birth to her daughter, I was 10 weeks pregnant. About two weeks after the birth, I went to visit her. I let myself in, snuggled down next to Kerry and her teeny-tiny brand new baby girl on the couch, and I unwrapped the two cheeseburgers I had brought for my snack.

"So," Kerry said, "which version of the labor story do you want to hear?"

"The real one," I said between bites. "Just tell me. I'll be fine."
In the spirit of solidarity, here is mine.

First Trimester: The Egg Lands!

The double blue line is so solid that I couldn't miss it if I were drunk, or visually impaired from crying over onions, or wearing sunglasses while biking at a high speed inside a pitch-black railroad tunnel. I'm definitely not drunk, and I haven't been for a long time, and I won't be for the next few years because I begin taking an occasional sip of alcohol again only when the 2020 pandemic hits. I also avoid cutting onions whenever possible, even if it means leaving them out of a recipe that desperately needs them. And although I have survived biking through a railroad tunnel in Montana blind because I forgot my sunglasses were on, I was not about to do any of that while peeing on a stick.

The test instructions say to wait two minutes, so I sit quietly on the toilet with my hands crossed and count the seconds as slowly as I can. However, I quickly revert to a child cheating at hide-and-go-seek: my counting speed increases to rapid fire at 62, then loses patience altogether. After a winged, totally inaccurate 88 seconds I sneak a peek at the top of the sink and can see from three feet away that the second blue line is even darker than the first. My results are so confident they don't even wait for their deadline.

My husband Jacob doesn't know about the test. I decided to purchase it today after some twists in yoga class made me feel like I was about to lose my lunch out of two orifices at the same time, and I fled the studio and headed to the nearest pharmacy. Jacob is on the couch downstairs in shorts, cruising his Twitter feed while sipping a Negroni. I'm about to transform him into a man who drinks seltzer water with a wife who gags at the smell of alcohol and demands cottage cheese, apple-smoked bacon and scrambled eggs, and then follows that with a cheeseburger and a chicken burrito.

We started toying with the possibility of pregnancy a few short weeks ago, which is the same amount of time I spent studying for my first midterm exam in ninth grade. So for all those ladies who skipped their school sex education class, or who never had one at all, or who trust their partners to take care of birth control, or who think that pregnancy is some miracle that happens only when you have sex at the perfect preordained time with a partner the universe has chosen for you, I am here to slash all of those beliefs with a samurai sword and inform you in the most loving way possible that you should expect to get pregnant the very first time you have unprotected sex. Of course, it may not happen, but we must all be cognizant of that. No matter the time, no matter the place, no matter the man. Consider yourself served with this age-old cautionary tale. Pregnancy is a prize you are more likely to win when you are ill prepared.

I call out to Jacob to help me in the bathroom. He sets down his cocktail and gallops up the stairs, probably wondering if I have stubbed my pinky toe on the tub or discovered a tiny insect that I am too much of a wuss to deal with myself. He enters the bathroom and, because I don't know what to say, I just nod in the direction of the sink and the stick.

"And ... THAT'S a baby!"

These are the award-winning words of Amy and Caleb, some friends who we learn are also pregnant the day after our urine wand wields its magic. During our double dinner date, from behind a mask of soup steam, I can somehow smell pregnancy on Amy like some people have great gaydar, or like Emily Blunt sees Tom Cruise has the power of the Omega in that movie where alien robots take over the Earth. I catch a whiff of pregnancy from across the table and then chase down our friends' secret with the aggression of a terrier let loose in a squirrel park.

"Ha!" I crow with glee as they acknowledge the truth.

"Our parents don't even know yet," Amy says. "Just the bus driver, and now you."

I offer no juicy information of my own in return. Like a sneaky pregnant ninja, I retreat to my smoothie and stay mum for the rest of the night.

I keep my mouth shut for five whole days until Jacob and I realize that our parents might like to hear the news. Well, not completely shut. The morning after the urine test, I have to call from work and relay the events of the week to the receptionist at BirthCare in Alexandria, Virginia, so I can make my first appointment.

"BirthCare and Women's Health," she answers.

"Yes, um, I'd like to schedule an exam as soon as possible."

"What type of exam? A well woman exam?"

At this point, I scurry out of my chair, past a dozen occupied cubicles, through a secure door and into a hallway. It's my first pregnant pause!

"Actually, I took a home pregnancy test," I whisper as I stab frantically at the volume button to quiet my cellphone.

"Okay. And was it positive?"

"Uhhhhh ... yeeeeeeeeees." I'm not sure why my tongue feels that so many extra letters are necessary.

"Well, in that case, you are going to need a longer appointment. How's Tuesday, September 11th?"

Whoa. No way. That is four weeks and five days in the future. How will I survive the suspense until then? I can't even wait one week between episodes of "Mad Men," for fear of what will happen to Joan.

"Could I get something sooner? I mean, just in case the home pregnancy test was wrong? Like, I don't want to walk around for a whole month thinking I'm pregnant if I'm really not, you know?"

"Mmm. I see. Was the home pregnancy test inconclusive?"

I am silent.

"Those tests are REALLY accurate. If you don't believe it, you can just take another one."

First the test, now the telephone. Every plastic device I touch wants to affirm my fertility.

"So ... you're pregnant!" the receptionist says. "See you on the 11th!"

"Great," I say. "Cool. And so until then — I mean, because I won't be seeing you guys for a while and I won't know what to do — I guess I'll just drink a lot of cocktails and smoke a lot of cigarettes."

"Yeah," the receptionist says, stone cold. "That's really funny."

That week, at just six weeks gestation, I am already ready to retire my pre-pregnancy bras. My breasts quickly become so enormous that I begin to wonder whether the baby is growing there rather than in my uterus. I wouldn't be surprised. The whole pregnancy thing is so sci-fi, anyway.

Along with new bras, I also purchase a giant noodle-shaped body pillow. It quickly becomes a third wheel in our bed, adored by me and tolerated by Jacob. At this point, I am no longer able to sleep on my belly, and the body pillow spoons my tender torso just right.

Second Trimester: More Food, More Questions, Less Sleep

For me, the first pregnancy is all crazy erect nipples and ravenous hunger. Eating constantly is necessary to stave off the nausea known in common parlance as "morning sickness," probably called so only because morning is a time when most people are hungry. For me, the sickness is not a side effect of the morning; it is a side effect of hunger. Thus, I come to believe that it should just be called "hunger sickness." Or how about just "hunger?"

"Eat crackers!" my mother-in-law reminds me on the phone.

Even in the oppressive summer humidity, my nipples stand at attention like a military salute as I hunt the urban territory around my office for beans, guacamole, turkey sandwiches with bacon, Greek yogurt, whole chocolate milk and cottage cheese. Then there is fatigue, like being drugged or collapsing after a climb up a mountain. Then a tender belly, like the aftermath of a series of jabs to the stomach.

I chat with women around town who craved pickles, strawberries, spicy chicken sandwiches, fish, gumdrops, sour candy, peanut butter sandwiches and Parmesan cheese. My own cravings begin and end with the bovine. Before pregnancy, beef was a rare presence in my diet. By the beginning of the second trimester, I crave cheeseburgers and milkshakes, and I give thanks every day to the cows that wrought them. I worship the divine goddess and mother of cows over and over again, and she is reincarnated in a never-ending circle of life to build my baby.

To ease nausea, I also crave ketchup, pickles, salads with vinaigrette and anything else with a vinegar base. The smells of coffee and alcohol become repulsive. Chocolate and sugar were once my best mates, but I've now expelled them from the inner circle and will not return their phone calls. My insatiable sweet tooth evaporates and is replaced by a fang with an endless lust for animal meat.

The BirthCare midwives have me keep a diary for three days to confirm that I am eating enough protein. Between the two containers of yogurt and peanut butter sandwiches I eat for breakfast, and the chicken burritos with black beans for lunch, I have sailed past my quota by the time I come home for supper. Gone are my younger days as an occasional vegetarian or a "seldom to never" eater of animals. I have become a carnivorous Viking raider, and chickens are a sacred sacrifice to help my family grow.

Meanwhile, the possibility that I will run out of food on an airplane becomes my own personal nightmare. When I travel to a best friend's wedding in Texas, I meet flight attendants who are so kind it makes me cry: They let me go to the tiny bathroom even though the "fasten seat belt" sign is on, and bring me cold, damp paper towels because they see me handling the barf bag like a sweaty thief on a heist. Despite their kindness, I must fly armed with three days' worth of snacks when traveling on domestic airlines. They feed their customers as though they are rationing for war, and not even the sweet mewling plea of a pregnant woman for a stale snack will soften their heartstrings.

"My only regret," one of Jacob's cousins says wistfully at a family gathering, "is that I didn't eat a hamburger before I went into labor." I take note to have one on hand at all times around my due date.

The second trimester brings us into childbirth class. In our Bradley Method class, my heart lightens when I hear that you can eat and drink water throughout your labor. If I need two sandwiches per hour for a car trip, heaven knows what I will need to drag myself through the marathon of birth.

Jacob does not enjoy this experience quite as much as I do. The first sign of disaster hits when he walks into the classroom and sees that there are no chairs; instead, we will be sitting for 12 weeks on yoga blankets and mats. Like many men who didn't grow up using squat toilets, Jacob has lost the ability to sit cross-legged on the floor for two hours without pain in his lumbar and despair in his heart.

Moreover, Jacob balks at every birth-related service not supported by scientific study. So, he Googles every service our teacher mentions on his phone to check facts. Childbirth is a business like any other, and there are many placebo effects you can buy with your money.

Bradley Method is geared toward preparing you for natural childbirth, but because we plan to deliver at BirthCare's birth center, I feel incredibly privileged because I don't anticipate major conflicts. BirthCare has a solid history of mother-centric natural childbirth. In general, I am empowered and the midwives will not do anything to my body without my permission. They will let me labor in whatever funky position I choose. They will let me be as involved or uninvolved as I want to be in catching the baby and cutting the umbilical cord after it stops pumping blood. They will give my baby and me valuable "skin to skin" time. They will not separate me from my baby for any reason. And they will let me do whatever I please with my placenta.

Instead of a sterile, cold, impersonal hospital environment with machines and background noise, the birth center is like a quiet, inviting home where you have your baby in a clean, well-equipped bedroom. The birthing rooms come complete with big comfortable beds, a Jacuzzi tub, soft chairs, a kitchen, huge bouncy balls to labor on and medical equipment gracefully hidden in the wardrobes.

At BirthCare, there is no Pitocin to induce labor, which is fine because I want to rely on my hormones. No epidural, which is great because I want to move like a monkey, and moving the way I want will help labor go better. The birth center's episiotomy rate is less than two percent, which is fantastic because I have a fear of sharp objects near my orifices. No C-sections, which is awesome because I don't want surgery. If Pitocin or a C-section become necessary, I can be transferred to a hospital 15 minutes away.

At my appointments, my midwives talk me step-by-step through all the decisions I need to make and give supportive guidance as my belly grows. I feel like I now have seven caring, wise new aunts with nursing degrees. The midwives pose questions such as:

"Are you planning a birth center birth or a home birth?"

"Do you have a birth plan?"

"What are you doing to prepare for childbirth?"

"Whom have you chosen as your birth assistant?"

"Have you pre-registered with the hospital in case you need to be transferred?"

Then they cheer with excitement as we listen to the baby's heartbeat, ask me how I feel, and administer warm, fuzzy words of comfort.

"Birth center birth or home birth?"

I decided on a birth center birth way back when Jacob and I were engaged. I knew I wanted to have children with Jacob, and I was scoping out places where childbirth looked merry. I also knew that a hospital birth wasn't my first choice — I just wanted a homier experience. On the other end of the spectrum, a home birth was out of the question for me, as our house was under major construction. When I was six months' pregnant, there were large portions of drywall missing and we washed dishes in the bathroom.

On my first visit to BirthCare, the midwives had me as soon as I saw oven mitts covering the stirrups on the exam table. They also engaged in real discussion. The midwife on duty that day spent a whole hour talking to me about my medical history, work life and family. She listened when I said I had a bad reaction to hormonal birth control and then reviewed my options. The midwives were upfront about which patients could give birth at the center, and which patients could not because they were too high-risk. They even asked questions about my relationship with Jacob, to make sure I felt safe and supported at home.

"Do you have a birth plan?"

In theory, this is a list of labor and postpartum options to discuss with your healthcare provider as well as your partner, in case your partner needs to advocate for you.

As it turns out, Jacob and I don't have a lot to discuss — not because we avoid confrontation, but because we happen to come from families that had similar beliefs about childbirth. Our mothers were breastfeeders and advocates of natural birth. Neither of our families practiced circumcision. Our mothers even quote the same dang books by Dr. T. Berry Brazelton.

In our childbirth class, Jacob and I — warm in our cocoon of like-minded coexistence — are reminded that other couples may need to compromise. One couple in our class has clearly never discussed circumcision before, and it suddenly emerges that the man is pro and the woman is anti.

"Whoa!" whispers Jacob, who delights in the juice of an awkward moment.

Then there are the various thoughts about what to do with a placenta. Some involve eating it in capsules or as an entree. One classmate's parents used it to grow a grove of apple trees, one tree over each of the spots where the placentas from the births of their three children are buried.

"Let me just say," jokes our classmate, "that the apples from my tree are better than my brother's."

I am grateful for engaging moments like these, because the truth is that I am hard-pressed to keep my pregnant brain awake until childbirth class wraps up at 9 p.m., much less compose a birth plan. When asked to draft a birth plan, I jot down two bullet points in my Bradley Method book, and then promptly resume the eating of snacks.

"So, what notes did you take for your birth plan?" the midwife asks at my next appointment.

"Just two things," I report. "Number one, no mirrors." That is, no mirrors so that I can watch the miracle of myself giving birth. There were mirrors once during a bikini wax, and it's just not my jam. "And number two: I do not want to do anything with the placenta." I'm not willing to pay good money to fuss with organs that can't be donated, and at the time, I was told that placentas could be donated only after a planned C-section. The prospect of eating my own organs brings me no joy, there are no known predators in the halls at BirthCare and we have plenty of protein to eat at home.

"What are you doing to prepare for childbirth?"

Ugh. Really?! Now that my workout options are limited, I literally dream about sprinting, jumping on trampolines and swinging like a gymnast on uneven bars. Meanwhile, my awake self is too pooped to party. Neither of these two versions of me are improved by the fact that I have pregnancy insomnia and cannot relax.

One night, I cannot get comfortable even with the help of that beautiful noodle-shaped body pillow that I ordered online during trimester one, and that has become an intractable addition to our marriage bed. I must have been tossing and turning, because our dog, Diggity, pops to a seated position and growls low at me, the first time she has ever growled in the direction of a human being who is not ringing our doorbell to deliver mail. As soon as she realizes she is awake and I am not a postal worker, she stops. She must have been having an amazing dream about a squirrel chase that I rudely interrupted. Then Jacob chimes in with his own commands to lie still.

"But I can't sleep," I whine through the dark, and my gentle husband barks at me for the first time in our seven years together.

"Well," he says, "you're not making it easier by keeping both of us up."

The best way to fall asleep is by leaning back against Jacob, with his legs on either side of me, Diggity cuddled at my feet and the baby kicking somewhere in the middle. Still, on New Year's Eve, we don't go out and I spend the night in tears. I am sitting in a home that I own with my husband who I am so happy to be having a child with and our adorable spotted terrier and yet I cry.

I cry for no reason, and because hormones have hijacked my life. I cry because I haven't slept well in weeks. I cry because after work, I no longer have an ounce of energy to do anything else. I cry because waddling around with a fetus taking over my internal organs isn't loads of fun. I cry because I am having an existential crisis, and life as I know it is about to change. In short, everything is about to turn itself upside-down and emerge head first through my birth canal.

To whip my weeping, sedentary self into shape for childbirth I attend my Bradley Method class, I practice yoga, I read a hypno-birthing book my friend Jessica mails me from Oregon, and I walk. My Bradley Method course equips me with practical knowledge about the physiology of labor. Yoga and hypnobirthing give me an arsenal of relaxation tools, coping skills and, for better or worse, razor-sharp self-awareness. On my walks I call lifelines like Michelle, my best friend from kindergarten, when I feel over-whelmed and want to walk into oncoming traffic.

Thanks to Bradley Method classes, I learn the science of hormones and what feelings to expect during the flow of labor. The acrobatic positions shown in our book also provide us with great entertainment.

But ultimately, the following is all Jacob ends up taking away from our 12-week course on childbirth:

1. He should wear a clean shirt to catch the baby in case I deliver in a car or before the midwife can reach us.
2. He should never, ever, under any circumstances try to push the baby back in.

Thanks to yoga, I stay limber. I strengthen my pelvic floor in preparation for labor. I maintain good posture even as the weight of the baby yanks my neck and shoulders forward. Despite the baby cramping my lungs, I breathe deep and align breath with movement, which will help with endurance for the upcoming marathon. Above all, I stay aware of my body so I will be able to make adjustments when the pain comes.

Through hypnobirthing and yoga nidra (yogic sleep) techniques, I learn to relax like a boss. I coexist with Jacob in bed once again. I rest in meditation and become a master at putting myself to sleep. I am now ready for my Broadway debut, if they can just find me a role as a character in a coma.

And that in sum is my childbirth curriculum.

"Have you chosen a birth assistant?"

BirthCare requires that you choose a birth assistant, which is sort of like a doula but someone who also has a ton of the medical training a nurse would have. Some birth assistants even have nursing degrees. Doula certification is part of their résumé, but birth assistants go far beyond that to become trained in CPR and neonatal resuscitation. They learn how to listen to fetal heart tones and assess maternal and infant vital signs, how to help stop a life-threatening hemorrhage, how to correct fetal distress, and so much more.

I send a mass email to all the birth assistants on their list. Lori is one of several who write back, and she says she is available in March. She is open because she wisely takes only two clients per month so that she is less likely to miss any of the births she has committed to assist. Lori has been a birth assistant for more than seven years and already has attended more than more than 250 births by the time I meet her. In addition to this work, she has three kids and a full-time day job, yet she still finds time to come to my local Ethiopian coffee shop on a weekend afternoon to talk.

Lori gives me a great hug and generously recounts all three of her birth stories — one happy hospital birth, one traumatic hospital birth and then an unpleasant but healthy birth at home. During our meeting, she impresses me as someone who has seen a variety of shows that childbirth has to offer, and is now professionally dedicated to helping other women have the births they want. So I invite her to assist with mine.

"Have you pre-registered with the hospital in case you need to be transferred?"

Yes. This takes just a few minutes online. Of course I hope for a perfect birth for which no hospital is needed, but I am humble enough to have a Plan B. Hope for the best, plan for the worst. After all, who knows what mood the bully dragon will be in the day my baby comes.

Third Trimester: Mama Bear Rears Her Head and Roars

Toward the end of pregnancy, I feel like a mother bear deep in hibernation. If provoked, I may emerge from my cave and attack. Rest is essential and patience is thin. Approach a pregnant woman slowly, or let her approach you. If she looks sleepy, back away quickly unless you come bearing food, drink or other gifts. Ask very little of her for the duration of winter.

The great score of maternity leave for the working woman is the relief that comes with finally sliding into home base and removing my shoes. I trot out of the office and head home to chug gallons of electrolytes, read a novel and take a nap. At long last, a reprieve from the professional paparazzi!

As one of many in a long line of American women who work outside the home until their due dates, I feel like I am on the field in front of a crowd for too long and am exhausted from the spotlights. Between the puppet mastery of prenatal hormones, hunger and a sudden Earth-shattering shift in personal priorities, every nuance of work life suddenly became superfluous. Previously, one could play the game of work with tolerance, good humor, patience and joy. The pregnant self rolls her eyes, bleeds inwardly from biting her tongue and fantasizes about throwing empty burrito bowls at the head of anyone who makes demands.

Sweet, simple questions such as, "What time is that meeting again?" prompt irrational fantasy dialogue from the pregnant self such as, "How the devil can you expect me to remember? Have you seen the size of this uterus?! I can take care of only one human being, and that human being is perched painfully atop my bladder as we speak. Now you must go while I eat hamburger."

A colleague asks, "Do you have a minute?" Suddenly, the pregnant self is wrapped in a vision in which she chucks a carton of chocolate milk in the air shouting, "Are you insane? I cannot indulge in speculation with you about the ownership of time. A baby's ass is in my rib cage! Now procure me another carton of chocolate milk with maximum fat content. That is all."

Maybe the pregnant self is really just a more transparent self. Or pregnancy is evidence that there is no self. Rather, it is evidence that all humans live every day gripping the reins on our wild, mustang hormones.

The last part of pregnancy is the true test of patience. I am waiting for a party, but I have no idea when that party will happen. I take long walks with my dog at a turtle's pace, and I stay well-hydrated and well-fed, because I know it will be the longest night of my life. But I don't yet know when that night will be.

How do you plan for an unplanned party? I start thinking that I won't leave the house for a couple of weeks because of a huge oncoming storm and an alien invasion, except that huge storm is happening in my uterus and that alien is the most beautiful child we will have ever seen. What should we stock up on while we wait this out?

Prep List for the Labor and Postpartum Party

1. Exercise ball to sit on if chairs become awkward

They do.

2. A vehicle so we can drive to BirthCare

Because we don't have a car, we need some sort of reliable vehicle in which I can let it all hang out in case I go into labor at four in the morning. Our friends Amy and Caleb are now sequestered with their own adorable newborn, so they kindly lend us their second car in advance of my due date.

3. Enough food to fill the freezer

Who wants to waste time cooking when a new baby is in the room? Because pregnancy has turned me into a rabid carnivore, we make a pot of beef stew with carrots and onions, red bean chili, spicy tomato sauce for shakshuka, and sauce for ragù alla bolognese. Then we divide our spoils into two-person portions and freeze them neatly in vacuum sealed bags.

4. Arrangements with loved ones to join in the effort

We book my mom for the first two weeks postpartum, and then my in-laws for Week 3. What's more, Jacob arranges to take off work to support me during the first couple of weeks after our parents depart.

5. Great television, podcasts, movies and books to entertain us

Just in case we get bored as we stare at each other waiting for the guest of honor to arrive.

Labor: The Party Starts

Now sit down next to me and I will tell you my labor story. I will tell you how I took all the pain and wrapped my body around it like a blanket. I will tell you how I dove with that pain down to its core, and found my baby there.

Our baby came out into the world on a cold, rainy night that burst into the first warm day of spring. It would be the last night I wore my winter boots that year. That morning, I had a breakfast date with Jacob downtown. I ate huevos rancheros. I could barely fit my belly in the chair and waddled downstairs every eight minutes to pee one tablespoon each time.

After breakfast, Jacob and I went for my mandatory 41-week ultrasound appointment and had a contraction. BirthCare requests an ultrasound at 41 weeks to look at the volume of amniotic fluid surrounding the baby. This scan gives a sense of whether the baby and placenta are healthy, and may help healthcare providers decide whether it is reasonable to allow another week of gestation.

I had already been having false labor contractions, or prodromal labor, on and off for about three weeks. So when a contraction hit me at 10:30 a.m. I lay nonplussed on my side under that sexy paper gown, my belly slick with gel, watching my white phantom baby pulse on the black screen. I didn't yet know which contractions were real or not real, so I thought nothing of that very first one.

After the ultrasound, I drove home in our borrowed car and had a contraction every 20 minutes behind the steering wheel. Then Jacob and I went for a spicy Indian lunch around the corner from home. Another pregnant woman was having lunch with her girlfriend at the next table, not nearly ready to pop but far enough along for my husband to congratulate her without risk of embarrassment. She asked me when my due date was. When I told her it had come and gone a week prior, her nose and top lip wrinkled into a grimace like a cute little pug.

"Is this your first?" she asked.

"Yes," I said. "But, you know, they say first-time moms are on average eight days late."

"Oh." She made the face again. Obviously, this was her first time hearing this information.

"Well," she said, her pug wrinkles dissolving into a hopeful smile, "maybe today will be the day!"

That afternoon, we had our weekly appointment at BirthCare. A couple in their mid-sixties were sitting on a couch in the lobby, their presence and age a telltale sign that a) they must have a daughter or daughter-in-law and b) said daughter or daughter in-law must be in the throes of labor upstairs. My appointment was less eventful, other than the mild contractions that continued throughout my exam. However, because it was week 41, our midwife, Elin, dictated the following plan:

Thursday (8 days late)
You will rest, watch movies, drink lots of water and eat well. Good times will be had by Katy. Jacob will be in the kitchen cooking.

Friday (9 days late)
You will go for a long walk, have sex, and then do some nipple stimulation. Good times will be had by all.

Saturday (10 days late)
You will take castor oil. Good times will be had by no one.

Sunday (11 days late)
You will come into the birth center for more induction-type things. No more good times will be had until the baby comes.

After the plan was hatched, we proceeded back downstairs, past the muted sounds of screaming through the walls separating exam rooms from birthing rooms. I paused like a voyeur in the hallway to listen.

"Yes," Elin said, "that is the sound of pushing. Let's move along now, move along!"

Jacob walked and I waddled to the car. I drove.

"Will you promise me something?" I asked Jacob.

"Yes."

"Please don't let me scream like those women in the movies."

At home, Elin's birth plan went into effect. In other words, I spent the afternoon reading "Gone Girl," by Gillian Flynn, relaxing on the couch and watching old episodes of "Mad Men." I took note that my contractions had continued at a pace all afternoon, consistently 12 to 20 minutes apart, but not increasing in intensity. We ate beef stew and I drank Gatorade. I took a warm shower, and cuddled into bed with my noodle-shaped body pillow between my legs at 9 p.m.

After that, shit got real.

Active Labor: When Shit Gets Real

Gil Fronsdal, a Buddhist teacher and scholar who lectures on Buddhism and meditation, recorded a 50-minute talk about dealing with pain. In that lecture, he distinguishes between objective and subjective sources of pain. For example, a nail in your forehead would be an objective source of pain. Of course, he says, if we can remove an objective source of pain that is harming our bodies maybe that's a good idea. I would agree: After all, why would we walk around with nails hurting our heads for no good reason? I sincerely hope that if Jesus of Nazareth were alive today and saw someone walking around with nails in his forehead, he would stand outside the temple and remove them and then call out everyone who was responsible for that abuse.

So to ease the objective source of the pain on my rainy night of labor, since I couldn't magically remove the baby from my body and I had decided not to use anesthesia in a hospital, I pulled these tools from my mental toolbox:

- Be mindful, present and hyperaware of your body. Notice when a contraction is coming and position yourself to face the pain. Follow each trace of sensation so you can predict what is about to happen, and watch it bravely like a warrior. If you face the pain instead of running from it, somehow it becomes a lot less scary.
- Lift pressure off the pain. For me, most labor pain was deep in the pelvic girdle, so lifting pressure was accomplished on my hands and knees with a neutral spine, which is often referred to in yoga as "tabletop" position. In tabletop, I let my

hands and legs support me, and completely relaxed around
my pelvic girdle. Meanwhile, for folks with back labor, I
have heard that relief might come from having hard pressure
placed on the small of the back. Learn your body well before
labor so that wherever pressure occurs, you can shift the rest
of your body to ease it.

- Let your body go. Above all, cede control of the pelvic girdle.
  Once labor hits, the time for Kegel exercises is officially
  over. It is time to let all those muscles RELAX. That night,
  I let bowel movements pass without any resistance. I wore
  a pad and lay towels on the floor so I could pee wherever a
  contraction hit. Labor is not a time for propriety. It is a time
  for shoving propriety out of the goddamn way so that the
  pregnant body can fulfill its mission.
- Relax your body between contractions. Treat relaxation like
  a job. As soon as a contraction began to subside, I started an
  inventory of every part of my body — my face, my jaw, my
  shoulders, my chest and all the way down to my feet and my
  toes — and one by one, I released any muscle or limb that
  felt tense. Just like I would turn off all the lights in my house
  at bedtime, I turned off all my muscles between contractions
  and put them to sleep.

However, in labor you can't just remove the objective source of the
pain like you can your hand from a hot stove. You have to hang
out with the pain, relax around it, and wait for it to pass you like a
semitruck on the street. When you cannot alleviate the objective
source of the pain you must cope by changing your subjective
experience, by finding a new response to the pain that comes ...
and comes ... and comes in waves that can knock you over.

Therefore, to change my subjective response to pain, these were
some of the words of comfort I gave myself throughout labor...

A gift from another mother in my childbirth class:

"You are SAFE, and your baby is SAFE."

(Even if you think something unsafe is happening, summon a lifeline and outsource the stress. Let no stress stay in your body during labor: Adrenaline will just stall labor and make it last longer. Treat your body like a little bunny that you are trying not to scare, because it has a very sweet and delicate heart.)

A gift from yoga:

"Find the ease in the effort."

(Ha! I like to think of this as a more poetic version of my mother saying, "Whether you like it or not, you're here now, so you may as well try to enjoy it." Think of labor as a crazy party where some horrible person spiked the brownies with psychotropic drugs and didn't tell you. Now you're tripping, and you really didn't want to be tripping, but there's nothing you can do about it, so you can at least try to have one fun hallucination.)

A gift from myself:

"Welcome the pain. It is here to help bring you your baby."

(Let the pain come in and do its job. Imagine the pain is a team of badass firefighters who want to get your baby out.)

A gift from my friend Amy:

"Just take it one contraction at a time."

(That's right. Don't try to be an overachiever. Just think of each contraction as the only painful thing you will ever have to conquer for the rest of your life. Don't let your mind wander and start thinking, "Holy Jesus, how long is this going to last and is it going to get worse and how am I going to make it through a bajillion of these?!" because thinking like that will only bring you down.)

A gift from the Persian Sufi poets:

"This too shall pass."

(Because it will, and when it does, the whole era of pregnancy and labor will shrivel into dust when stacked up next to the infinite pride and joy you will soon experience as a parent.)

A gift from my mother-in-law:

"Just remember that no matter how bad things get, at the end of the day you get to take home that baby!"

(And taking home the baby is the AWESOMEST thing EVER!!!!!!!! The sum total of all gifts you've ever received since your own birth will seem TOTALLY LAME in comparison!!!!!!!!)

And when all else failed, a gift from kindergarten:

Count. Pick a number and think to yourself, "Okay, when I reach the number X, this contraction will be over! One, two, three, four …"

I slept between the harder contractions until after midnight. I would relax and sleep for a few minutes, then stiffen against the body pillow when the pain came. Then I would shuffle to the bathroom to empty my bowels or my bladder. Finally, I would return to bed, where Diggity was perturbed that I had interrupted her slumber. I would crawl back under the covers and conjure images of myself sleeping on the floor of a quiet temple, or on the warm sand of a beach, or in a meadow with a light wind brushing along the tips of the grass. These were the happy places I took from meditation sessions, yoga nidra, and glorious nights spent on the beach, in the mountains and desert, or anywhere I had ever slept well.

Yet sometime after midnight I lost my grace, became significantly less ladylike and migrated permanently to the bathroom. There was no poop left for my body to expel, but there was still pee, every time my uterus contracted. How do I know my husband is amazing? Because he said, "Just pee the bed, sugar. Who cares?" But I didn't. I truly regret that. I missed my one big chance to pee the bed and still be loved.

In the bathroom, I spent several hours laboring on my hands and knees atop a thick, comfy towel I laid on the tile floor, and it really did help take the pressure off my pelvis. Finally, by about 4 a.m., my contractions were five minutes apart. I was also dripping fresh blood onto the floor with each one. My voice separated from my body, and it told Jacob that he should call the midwife. (Remember: Outsource stress. Don't scare the baby bunny.)

"She wants to talk to you," Jacob said, and he put the phone on speaker atop the toilet tank.

"I … can't," I groaned. This is the clever ploy of midwives: They force you to talk so they can gauge how functional you are. If you can say pretty words on the phone like a lady, then you're not nearly far enough along. If you sound like a zombie, or a dying primate, or maybe Mickey Rourke after his heart attack in "The Wrestler," then they can feel confident that they won't be wasting their time if they tell you to come in.

"Hey, Katy," Elin's voice said from the toilet. "How are you feeling?"

I grunted my greeting like the zombie I now was. "Ehhhhhhh!"

Silence.

"I just had a contraction," said the zombie version of me.

More silence.

"Do you know how far apart they are?" Elin asked.

"Ehhhhhhhh." That's zombie for "very goddamn close together." However, zombies, like pregnant people, tend to lose track of time.

"I just had a contraction."

More silence.

"I just had another contraction." And so on.

"Okay," Elin said. "I think it's time to come to the birth center."

Jacob helped me move from nakedness into my baggiest skirt and a T-shirt and asked me to put on my boots, which I could not imagine doing because it involved bending over a giant, contracting uterus. I had gone to a salon the week before and had the rare treat of a pedicure, so that no matter how ugly other body parts became, I could stare at those twinkly toenails that were painted bright gold. But right then, I was thinking of taking those gorgeous feet out into the rainy night and scuffing them up on some gravel to avoid the horror of a mid-shoe contraction.

Somehow, Jacob got my boots on. Then my coat was on, too, and I walked backward down the stairs on my knuckles like a gorilla. I had a contraction on the stairs, a contraction in the front hall, a contraction on the porch. I had a contraction standing on the street in the rain with my hands planted on the hood of the car. I stared down the front passenger seat, eyed the dreaded seat belt like an enemy and formed a strategy for occupation. Then, at about 4:30 a.m., Jacob drove me to the birth center as I knelt backward in the front passenger seat, embracing the headrest with my chin on its shoulder.

We arrived at BirthCare by 5 a.m.. I looked no one in the eye. I was totally focused on my body, surveilling it for signs of the next contraction. It was still dark. I remember the hood of Jacob's yellow raincoat. My hair was damp and somehow, against all odds, pulled back with an elastic band. Lori and Elin were waiting for us, and that made me feel as though nothing could go wrong, because they would be able to handle anything. Elin was a voice in the dark hallway of the birth center, with pants and sleeves that felt soft when I leaned against her. But I stayed with my body, watched and listened, and somehow knew what I had to do. Then I got down on all fours, and climbed the stairs on hands and knees so my legs and arms could take the pressure when the contractions hit.

"And that," Elin said, "is a totally legitimate way to go up stairs."

In the birthing room, Elin somehow managed to perform a vaginal exam despite my refusal to lie on my back and found that I was already seven centimeters dilated; in other words, in the transition phase of labor, about 70 percent of the way until pushing could begin. Hallelujah, Mother of God, Allah is merciful and Jesus is Lord! I remember thinking that if I were still only a measly centimeter or two dilated after that much pain, there was no way in the burning flames of hell I was going to survive labor without medication. But I had already survived it. I was rounding the final curve in the track. I was in the home stretch. I could see the finish line.

Reinvigorated, I mounted a bouncy exercise ball Elin had set out — my new throne — and I labored sitting on a Chux pad laid over the top of the big ball. I exhaled fully each time until my lungs felt empty and then inhaled deeply to fill them up again. Just before each contraction hit, I rose and planted my hands on whatever was there — the bedpost, Elin's knees, the side of the bathtub. Between contractions, I sucked Gatorade out of a straw, let myself pee the huge pad and rested. Always, in between contractions, I turned off all the lights in my body's house and rested. My birth assistant gently leaned forward in the dark and pushed my shoulders away from my neck, her sweet touch a reminder to relax every corner of my laboring body. I told myself over and over that the pain would pass. I saw myself taking the baby home when the night was over. I imagined the baby safe inside my womb and the amniotic bubble, waiting patiently to be born.

Then my body shifted and switched gears. Instead of contracting, my muscles clearly pushed out, bearing down and racing like I was about to take the biggest poop of my life. Progress! Suddenly, the contractions felt productive, euphoric as my body flooded with oxytocin and endorphins. It felt like the warmth that bursts during a hard workout when your body is in the zone, or the pitched rolling of an ecstatic drug high, or the craze that flows through your body right before an orgasm.

At this point, Elin observed that I had progressed from dilation contractions to pushing contractions and asked me how I wanted to be. Again, I centered all attention on my body to decide what I needed to be comfortable. I mounted the bed and got on my hands and knees, with the exercise ball supporting my head and chest. Elin and Jacob were somewhere behind me. I waited for my body to bear down again and when it did, primal moans like a grizzly bellowing emerged low and unhinged from my mouth like nothing I had ever heard from a human. Oh my god. Who the hell was I becoming now?

"Take that sound," Lori murmured in my ear, "and send it straight to your bottom."

The next time my body bore down, I did just that. I harnessed my roaring voice and let it sing through my torso. I empowered the energy of my breath to push the baby. With each mammalian moan came hot pain isolated around my perineum, and the high of hormones rolling through my body around it. It was the "ring of fire" I had read about in childbirth class, heralding the arrival of the baby's head. After each exhale, I said one holy word — "Gatorade" — and Lori stuck the colored straw between my teeth. Meanwhile, Elin, Lori and Jacob met each exhale and bearing down with the oddly calm, civilized praise of a massage therapist watching a rugby match. "That's the way..." cooed Elin and Lori's soft, kind voices. "Great progress, Katy. Good work."

It went on. I felt as though only the power of purple Gatorade stood between me and a coma of total exhaustion. In my mind, the whole universe dissolved into one moment, and one contraction, and one sip of liquid, and one breath against the exercise ball on my bare chest. For everyone else, there could be past and future, but for me, there was only present. Somewhere out in the world, the night had ended and the sun had risen, but for me, my birth canal was the center of the universe. Finally, after one contraction, I heard Elin say, "Wow! Look at all that hair!" and I knew my baby's head was coming. After another contraction, I felt a burst of fiery sensation and a pop, as my baby's head broke the amniotic sac. Then hands and more pressure, as Elin reached in to check whether the umbilical cord was around the baby's neck. Then a mass slipping out of me like a seal sliding off a rock. And then, somewhere on an adjacent planet that was twirling and spinning in my direction, Jacob reached out and caught our baby.

"It's a boy," I heard someone say. The pain that had overwhelmed me for so many hours departed. I let my chin drop down to my sternum. I let my body shake to release the stress, and cried. After the tremors had run their course, I looked down through my shoulders and saw my son.

And then, there was another person in the room.

The baby next to me, cuddled against my chest. Skin to skin, the sweet way babies and those who bear them are meant to be. We stared at each other, the umbilical cord still pulsing. Jacob behind him with wet eyes. So much work to move my baby such a short distance.

We lay together like that for a while. It was daylight now. Lori and Elin took care of business in the background — weighing and measuring the baby, ordering the birth certificate and writing a record of the birth, cleaning up the birthing room and bathroom. Jacob rose to feed everyone the lasagna he had brought. We hadn't planned on the meal being breakfast.

"Your mom texted," Jacob said. "She asked if you took your walk yet. I wrote back, 'No, we had a baby instead. Mother and son are resting comfortably.'"

Marsha, one of the original founders of BirthCare, came into the room to congratulate us. She was opening the office to start the day's business. Small gears still turning as planets collide.

Three hours, two baby footprints, one slow shower and one quick family photo later, we were given instructions to go home and rest. After she helped me take my shower, Lori dressed me down to my shoes and walked me to the car. The sun shone. The baby slept. Jacob drove.

Ah, fresh air on my face through the open car window. The absence of pain. A feat accomplished. I called my mom, who was already en route to fly to us. Then I called my grandmother.

"Are you happy?" she asked.

I hope, for every parent's sake, that they have as much difficulty as I did answering this question because their happiness is as unbearable as mine.

First 30 Days Postpartum: Hard Poops and Happiness

There is so much literature out there to prepare for labor and birth. However, rarely do parents receive the same level of training for the aftermath. Thus, I prepared a list of two dozen essentials that served us during our first 30 days outside the womb together.

To comfort the person who gave birth:

1. Ibuprofen for pain relief

In the minutes after Enzo was born around 8 a.m., I felt no pain at all. Why? I was sky-happy high on endorphins and adrenaline. Thanks to the pixie dust of natural hormones, I was alert and attentive as Enzo cuddled next to me, warmed by my skin, the two of us still attached by our umbilical cord. After the cord stopped pulsing its valuable blood from the placenta, the midwife clamped and cut it, and I delivered the huge steak that was my placenta without even knowing it popped out. The birth assistant set Enzo on my belly and he shimmied his mouth up to latch onto my nipple. The midwife applied a dab of local anesthesia and gave me one or two small stitches I never felt as I cozied up, ecstatic, with my shiny new son. As Enzo was weighed and measured by the midwife and his daddy, I went to the toilet and shower with aid from the birth assistant. She then helped me get dressed, and I gushed over Enzo and our wonderful birth. By 11:30 a.m., three hours after Enzo entered the world, Jacob drove us home as Enzo slept in his new car seat and I felt fabulous. Tired, but fabulous. I took a luxurious nap all afternoon and was laughing when I woke up to my brother-in-law's arrival. I was giddy when my mom flew in that night.

Then, at some point, the adrenaline wore off and the pain set in. Nipple aches from the first days of nursing, pelvic aches from the birth, random muscle aches in my neck and back and legs and shoulders. Labor is hard work, and it felt like a muscle hangover after an insane marathon boot camp workout. There will be pain, so why not have some pain relief on hand?

2. Lots of water, plus vitamin C or magnesium or any other stool softener

It is a truth universally acknowledged that our first postpartum poops can hurt a lot. I didn't poop for several days after childbirth, and the first time I did, it was a little scary. It felt as though any pressure inside my pelvic area sparked tiny memories of labor, but without the happy hormones or the baby to anticipate. BirthCare midwives and my birth assistant had warned me about poop trauma, but in all the baby excitement, I had forgotten until it was time for the first poop. Before the next one, I chugged lots of water with vitamin C.

3. Heavy-flow maxi pads for postpartum bleeding

Just prepare as you would for a long, heavy period. For the first few days, I slept with Chux pads in the bed, courtesy of my midwives, and wore thick maxi pads during the day. I got enough maxi pads to last at least two weeks. I had heavy bleeding for only the first week postpartum; however, on Day 13, I did go to the bathroom and hatch one more surprise — a dollop of blood the size of an egg yolk.

From my midwives' 24-hour answering service, I learned that this red yolk probably came from the spot in my uterus where my placenta had been implanted. As the uterus ingeniously shrinks after childbirth, that spot sloughs off like a scab so your uterus can make itself good as new again and produce as many placentas as your family planning requires. Most child bearers are still bleeding more heavily than I was by the time this "scab" comes out, so they don't even notice. Just another sci-fi bit of childbirth that is totally normal.

4. Medline "cleansing bottle" (also called a "peri" bottle) to squirt warm water on yourself while you pee

Peeing can burn for the first week or two after childbirth. I kept that bottle in the bathroom and filled it with warm water — not too hot, not too cold, just like the porridge in "Goldilocks and the Three Bears." I would squirt myself just as I sat on the toilet and kept it going until pee time was over. My birth assistant said it best: "The warm water just makes your pee less 'burny.'"

Eight days after Enzo was born, my friend Kerry was standing outside the bathroom with him after she had changed his diaper like the champion she is. She spotted the cleansing bottle on top of the toilet and recalled its purpose immediately. "Ohhh," she said with compassion and a sisterly smirk, "I feel so bad for you!"

5. Wet wipes or soft washcloths to clean yourself after any business in the bathroom

Your skin can really hurt down there, and rubbing toilet paper on any privates may be an unnecessary evil. Besides, if you don't go through all of the wipes, you can always use them to clean your baby.

6. Lactation consultant

"I've seen worse," the BirthCare midwife on duty said when she saw my breasts two weeks postpartum. "But this makes me sad." I had scabs on my right nipple and bruises around both. She ordered me to stay topless as much as possible for a week to keep my nipples dry, and strongly recommended that I call a lactation consultant to prevent further injury.

The lactation consultant burst into our house like Mary Poppins, except that instead of a carpet bag she had a small suitcase containing antibacterial and antifungal ointments, nipple shields and a scale to see how much milk the baby was getting with each feed. She made me demo my nursing as I lay down on the bed, as I sat up, as I reclined on the couch, on my left side, on my right, and in several other acrobatic positions. Then she weighed Enzo each time to make sure my milk pipes were functioning properly. After two hours in her care — even with my wounds still there — breastfeeding was blissfully painless. It made me want to dance on chimneys and fly a kite.

In hindsight, I should have had a lactation consultant visit as soon as my milk came in on Day 2. Instead, I learned the hard way after three silly weeks spent screaming, crying and dreading every feeding because of sore, scabbed nipples from a latch that wasn't deep enough, bruises from my baby's mouth, and shoulder spasms from sitting in terrible postures. Immediately postpartum, my midwife and birth assistant had asked me repeatedly whether breastfeeding was going okay and advised me to request a lactation consultant if it wasn't. I guess I just thought the pain was normal.

Breastfeeding should not be that painful. If it hurts, something is probably wrong. And with so many things women do, breastfeeding is not always as easy and graceful as we may make it look. So, if there is pain, spring for a lactation consultant right as you start nursing. Your health insurance may even cover this service. That way, you can spare yourself all my misery, self-doubt and feelings of failure.

7. Something to protect your nipples as they adjust to the overstimulation they will receive as they transform into a 24/7 milk vending machine

During the first few weeks, I occasionally wore "nipple shells" under shirts when I still had scabs. Then, after my nipples healed, I switched to cotton breast pads or small cotton washcloths that I would stuff in my bra, then wash and reuse. With these two items, you will score twofold: You will neither chafe your sore nipples nor leak breast milk in public. Unless, of course, that's what you're into.

8. Nipple cream

This I spread all over my nipples as soon as I started nursing. I tried a bunch of brands given to me by other new mothers, who all had their favorite. I liked Lansinoh, because it's really substantial and doesn't melt off. I was also a fan of Burt's Bees nipple cream. Or if you want something all natural, try coconut oil.

9. "Milk saver," or some other device to collect milk that drips from the unused breast as you nurse

You may leak a lot of breast milk the first few weeks, and you may as well put it to good use, instead of just letting it drip onto your baby's head. I filled Enzo's first bottle from just a few days of leakage I collected. Then I went away for a few hours, got a dental cleaning and a massage, and I let his daddy feed him a bottle.

10. Electric breast pump with milk storage bags

In the United States, thanks to the Affordable Care Act (aka Obamacare), health insurance companies must now provide new mothers with some sort of breast pump. Call yours to find out what it offers. For hands-free pumping, you can also accessorize with a pumping bra so you can read, eat or operate the TV remote during milk factory operations.

11. If you like, some sort of cloth to cover yourself while you breastfeed in cold weather, or in front of any folks you would prefer not see you topless

I lost all hope of propriety within the first 30 days, because the same week my BirthCare midwife ordered me to remain topless was the week my in-laws were coming to stay. My father-in-law saw me topless. My brother-in-law saw me topless. During the first 30 days, the baby needs to eat at least every two hours, so unless you want to be antisocial, you just have to nurse in front of your people.

On this topic, my feminist husband would like to add, "You are not just breastfeeding in public for you: You breastfeed in public to make it easier for the parents who come after you!"

And my friend Amy would also like to add that it's entirely legal to breastfeed in public. All 50 states, the District of Columbia and Puerto Rico have passed legislation that either allows women to breastfeed in any public place, or at least exempts them from prosecution for indecent exposure. So feed your baby wherever you need to. If anyone has a problem with it, you can ask them whether they prefer a screaming baby or a quiet one. And if anyone tells you to breastfeed in a restroom, you can ask them if they would like to eat their lunch next to a toilet.

12. Someone to cook ALL your meals, do ALL your grocery shopping, and clean up after you and your baby 24/7 for at least two weeks, but preferably three to four

This is not just advice for prima donnas: Childbirth is serious physical exercise and trauma that demands equally serious recovery. Your pelvis hurts. Your butt hurts. Your boobs hurt. You need the kind of hydration and nourishment normally demanded by marathon runners. You can't really sit on your pelvis without cushions for at least two days, you are not supposed to walk far for the better part of a fortnight, and you may be needing maxi pads for up to six weeks. Your abdominal muscles are flopping off to the sides like a pillow, where pregnancy left them as the uterus took over your torso. Would you expect someone recovering from major surgery to cook and clean for herself? Alrighty then. Find some loved ones who understand the situation and you will see that they are more than happy to make themselves useful. And I mean useful. Don't invite anyone over who is going to expect YOU to entertain THEM, or who just wants to hold the baby while there is laundry to be done. Be clear that this assignment includes grocery shopping, cooking, washing dishes, doing laundry and anything else that most of us who aren't millionaires normally don't have the money to outsource.

13. A good book, podcasts, shows, games, or good company to add to the fun while you are breastfeeding or homebound

To comfort the baby:

1. Swaddles

The Aden + Anais brand of muslin swaddles were our favorite. They came highly recommended from my friends and co-workers and received accolades from the grandmas. They are gauzy (good for baby's temperature) and stretchy (good for swaddling) and they feel great on your baby's skin. Also look up a good video or demo on swaddling techniques so you learn to wrap them nice and tight. Enzo loved to be swaddled — once he started to smile, he would grin as we wrapped him.

2. Any lightweight baby carrier that frees your hands

These carriers are a win-win — the baby is happy to be close to you, and you are happy because your hands are free. The Moby enabled our first urban outings and the Ergo is what I used to carry Enzo through the airport, etc. However, like purses and luggage, there are a zillion good types. To each her own.

3. Front-snap shirts

With shirts that snap in the front, you won't have to pull anything over your baby's head or have to change clothes every time he gets himself wet or overshoots the diaper. Your newborn doesn't need fancy clothes, and babies grow so fast that it's not worth the money to buy them. Believe me, for the first few weeks, your baby will be wearing only a diaper, a shirt or a swaddle, and staying close to you. If it is cold, he will just need a warmer swaddle or more baby blankets. After the first few weeks, the best outfits are onesies that snap on the bottom and also have a wide neck and clever little shoulder creases so you can pull it down over the baby's shoulders in case it gets pooped on.

4. Comforting sound

In the quiet world outside your body, the lack of noise can be confusing. Shushing really comforts your baby, but shushing with your voice may get old fast. Hence, you may appreciate having some sort of repetitive, loud rhythmic sound to help your baby sleep. I found ocean waves and water sounds more pleasant than traditional white noise, but a lot of folks prefer the latter.

5. A chair that rocks (either a rocking chair for you both, or a bouncy seat for the baby)

Rocking helped soothe Enzo to sleep. However, I lacked the physical stamina during those first weeks to rock him with my body. Plus, rocking chairs make me motion sick. I received a secondhand bouncy chair (also called a bouncy seat) from Jacob's aunt, and it provided me with divine, handsfree time until Enzo was old enough to roll over.

6. Pacifiers

Have a couple on hand in case your baby — like ours — is comforted by sucking and you don't want your nipple to be used for comfort, because you are already giving out your nipples for food. Of the pacifiers we received, we liked the ones that had a little curvy bit that fit in Enzo's mouth just right.

7. Loads of diapers

In fact, shitloads of diapers. Newborns go through eight to 10 per day. Among the disposable diapers, our favorites were the ones with the line that turned a different color when Enzo was wet. Thanks to this handy line, you don't have to reach in and possibly dirty your hand checking the diaper. To limit our garbage output, we switched to cloth diapers after eight or 10 weeks, as soon as Enzo was big enough to wear them comfortably.

8. Really, really soft and absorbent washcloths

Get two dozen (or chop up a few larger soft pieces of fabric into two dozen pieces) if you wash laundry every two or three days, or fewer if you do laundry more often. They are essential for cleaning poopy baby bums and for gently cleaning your baby's skin. Like cloth diapers, we opted for washcloths over disposable wipes in an attempt to be sustainable.

9. Diaper wipe warmer

I am sure you don't like cold things on your bum, and neither does your baby. This clever little device immediately eliminated crying during diaper changes. It keeps your little baby washcloths steamed, warm and wet so you can just whip them out for pleasant diaper changes or a quick baby sponge bath. Plus, this way you don't need to dry your washcloths — just take them from the washing machine and return them to the steamer.

10. Arterial thermometer

This is essential if you want to take your baby's temperature without entering any orifices. We sent my brother-in-law out to get one on Day 2 postpartum when we realized how hard it was to take a crying baby's temperature with a regular thermometer.

11. Baby bottles

With bottles on hand, your baby can still eat if your own milk vending machine is temporarily indisposed for one of the following reasons: a) you had to go to a doctor's appointment, b) you are passed out exhausted at 4 a.m. and feel like waking up to breastfeed would push you over an edge, c) you need to make a phone call to someone who doesn't understand that newborns don't respect the artificial time constraints our modern society has imposed on us, d) you are dealing with an especially long and painful postpartum poop in the bathroom, or e) none of the above, but something that is equally dire or important.

All that being said, parenthood is truly awesome in a way that I could never have foreseen or fathomed. There is absolutely nothing else like it. It is pure joy, rewarding work and intense love with all the whipped cream and sprinkles and cherries in the world on top. And for every sleepless night, there are baby coos and giggles and first steps and a bond that opens a reservoir of love in our hearts that may overflow and flood the Earth. May you have a lifetime of these days. Enjoy the adventure.

Second Birth: Labor Like a Warrior

The second story will not be the same as the first. We fast-forward in time, to a new pregnancy. At the supermarket, I take the test in a bathroom stall, because I cannot wait eight blocks to get home. I watch the little white plastic window for signs. Once again, two lines.

It's Thanksgiving, and I don't drink wine with my friends and family. Not because a small glass of wine would make any real difference to my baby, but because of the nausea I feel when I smell alcohol. No one takes note of this. If you are a woman, no one cares what you are drinking or not drinking until they learn your body is producing human growth hormone. Then the transvaginal judgment begins.

This time, there is no explosion of excitement. Two and half years after my first child was born, nine weeks after a miscarriage, and 31 days after my last period, I am cautious with optimism. Joy will grow with the body of evidence.

Over the next few weeks, that evidence trickles my way. Exhibit A: drop-dead fatigue. I can no longer join Enzo for dance parties to Disney soundtracks. Instead, I come home from work, lie on the couch, watch him and feel guilty. Exhibit B: hunger. Bagel sandwiches with egg and cheese, piles of Greek yogurt, more chicken burritos, more cheeseburgers, plus all the ice cream, doughnuts and cookies I can lay fingers on. Exhibit C: a strong heartbeat on the Doppler when I visit the midwives. All three are proof that the baby is growing. Healthy, viable, strong. Bring it on.

This time, there will be no childbirth classes. I have misplaced my Bradley Method book and I don't even bother looking on our bookshelves to find it until weeks after the birth as I write this sentence.

The only pregnancy book I read is "Expecting Better," by Emily Oster. Every chapter shoots darts at another pregnancy myth, reviews literature on the topic and then sees where the dart lands. As I educate myself about pregnancy risks I write some terrible haikus to summarize what I have learned:

Smoking's bad, so bad
with babies, without babies
so clearly, always.

A drink may be fine
if you are sipping wine but
please, no hard liquor.

Enjoy deli meat.
Y'all just steer clear of cold cuts
with listeria.

You can drink coffee.
It won't hurt your baby but
you might gag. It smells.

Sushi? You love it.
Waddle where there's yummy fish
and no mercury.

The week I finish the book's sushi chapter, I walk out of my office and see a food truck selling maki, which I view as a sign from God. I eat salmon hand rolls for the rest of my pregnancy and never look back. My friend Amy, a nurse practitioner whom you may remember from my first birth story, hears this news and texts countless exclamation points at me for not discussing it with her previously. She enjoyed sushi responsibly starting with pregnancy number one.

This time, there are even more new bras. My chest is exploding and pounding with the pain of my pregnant breast size. At the

Breastfeeding Center in Washington, D.C., I am fitted by a lovely young saleswoman who introduces me to bra sizes I never even knew existed. I try on a DD cup, then an E, then keep singing the alphabet song until we hit the right letter. Three-year-old Enzo opens the curtain, goes back out again and tells the saleswoman I need a bigger one.

This time, there will be less yoga. I manage two yogic sleep workshops during the first trimester. After that, I do make it to a free class on Sundays, which I attend only after I have eaten four pieces of buttered toast with several eggs. As my belly grows, I fall from every pose. I am five foot two with a celestial belly and moon-size breasts wobbling into the railings and the walls. Our yoga teacher, a slender man with long hair and a soft mustache, quietly moves some things aside so I can grab a railing or a wall when my uterus and chest thrust me sideways. I rock back and forth, a tree uprooted in the wind. A leaning tower of baby.

I continue to walk three miles every day between work and home. During the first trimester, I also attend physical therapy sessions with a wonderful woman who massages muscle cramps that have been chronic since I gave birth two and a half years earlier. Every week, she digs her elbow into my right butt cheek and beats it into submission until the knots relax. She gives me a daily exercise regimen to strengthen my core muscles and stop the spasms. Almost every day, I do gentle strengthening for my abdomen and quadriceps, then stretch my side body and IT bands. When pelvic pain sets in from the baby weight, I do Kegel exercises like a series of prayer beads. My body stays healthy, maybe even evolves, as it softens into another pregnancy.

This time, there are no emotional roller coasters. I know the great reward that awaits me after these 40 weeks of work. I have chosen a new job with a slightly reduced schedule, knowing that another baby was on the way. I make choices that will not drive me to a tipping point. It's hard enough not to fall over as it is.

This time, there is one less mystery. It's a girl. With Enzo, because Jacob and I chose to leave his gender unknown, we also chose a girl name. Now we are parents and too tired to think of two names, so we go for the gender reveal at the 20-week ultrasound. However, the baby — who has been a prolific kicker up to now — has crossed legs at the exam as an act of protest. The technician, who is clearly terrified at the prospect of disappointing me, asks me to massage my belly and coerce movement. So I roll from my back to my left side. From my left to my right. Right back to left. Left back to right. We take breaks. The clock ticks. We start the game over, roll back and forth and round again. After the better part of an hour, there is still no reveal. The baby keeps legs and ankles pretzeled together like strands of a vine. Everywhere, there is translucent ultrasound slime.

"It's okay if I don't find out," I say finally. "Really. It's not a big deal."

"No!" the technician cries. She looks me in the eye, the Doppler in one hand, and shakes it like a judge in scrubs wielding a gavel. "I'm not letting you leave here until you know!" She spreads yet more goo, the tube gripped with purpose. The ultrasound has now gone on so long that I have seen every other part of my baby's body four times. There is a beautiful heart with its proper chambers, all 10 fingers and toes and perfect proportions. But I feel as though I've been at a show for too long and the excitement has worn off. It's time to go home.

Then she shouts, "It's a girl!" It is. I can see the little black space between my baby's pelvic bones on the screen. That's it — that's all we've got. The technician is so pleased. But am I? My first feeling is fear. What will I do with a daughter? I can't imagine. I live in a country where women are occasionally treated as equals but it's also 2016, and misogyny is rampant. The Republican presidential nominee is boasting about sexual assault. Even rape is still not taken seriously in some courts and schools. Basic access to birth control and sex education is opposed by conservatives. Churches are preaching that women should be obedient to their husbands. I sigh, and shed a few tears that the technician doesn't see. There is a lot of work to do to raise our daughters up. Now that work is mine, too.

Moreover, during the last months of pregnancy it dawns on me that I will soon be in labor for a second time, and that I cannot outsource that job to someone else. I've got a daughter coming. I need to begin practicing some radical responsibility.

To prepare for this second labor, I practice relaxing body parts one by one. During my low-intensity physical therapy regimen I focus on the discomfort and try to enjoy it, find the ease in the effort. I remind myself that labor is just about coping with pain — pain that will pass, pain that brings with it an adorable new baby. Just a few days more effort for a lifelong reward.

I collect all the home birth supplies that BirthCare recommends and has summarized on a one-page list. At 37 weeks, my new birth assistant Holly comes to the house to check my preparations. Since we are planning a home birth this time, I shouldn't have to ride in a car during labor, and if you read my first labor story, you may recall that for me this is phenomenal. The inventory I am advised to stock at home totals more than 40 items, including an oxygen tank with a mask and tubing, cleaning supplies to remove blood and other bodily fluids, food and liquids, a collection of basic first aid tools, and things to keep the baby warm after birth. Some things on the list cost nothing, including "a quiet place for the CNM and birth assistant to lie down" if labor goes long. Many items are already on hand, such as garbage bags, ice, paper towels and washcloths. There are even helpful instructions on how to make up my bed so that childbirth doesn't destroy the mattress.

"Well, you seem prepared but relaxed," Holly says with a tone of approval. She checks the supply inventory in my closet, and tests the oxygen tank I borrowed from BirthCare. She asks me questions including, "How will you heat up blankets to keep the baby warm?" "Where should the midwives take turns resting if labor goes long?"

She tours the house so that she can find what she will need for the birth. My prenatal hormones feel whatever the opposite of prepared is, but I do have everything on the list. And if that is all the experts say is needed, then I will trust that until further notice.

Finally, I pre-register at a preferred hospital just in case I need to be transferred, and map out the distance by car. Less than 20 minutes.

Then comes the humid heat of summer, with record-high temperatures. It is the worst time of the year for my abdomen to be a space heater. I hobble home from work, melting like a sad crayon in my maternity dresses. I switch into flip flops at work, because shoes are too much. I want to strip to my underwear and be covered in ice. I regret not living in the western fjords of Iceland. I want to give birth on a glacier while the Arctic breaks across my back.

Then comes sickness. At 39 weeks, there is congestion in every sinus that drains into my chest. I stand in front of the air-conditioning unit in our bedroom and gasp for air. I learn to be content with shallow breaths and not to inhale any deeper, because the effort is fruitless. My birth plan that week is to go straight to the hospital when contractions start, or to inhale all the oxygen from the tank in my closet and see what that's like.

Then I go to my 39-week ultrasound and my amniotic fluid is low. Almost too low. It's dipping below seven percent and my baby is measuring underweight on the ultrasound, possible signs that she is not thriving. Or the baby is just fine, and I am severely dehydrated from the hellish climate in which I am gestating. The radiologist tells me I will need another ultrasound in a week to follow up. I relate this news to the midwives, and they tell me to drink more than 100 ounces of liquid per today to try to boost my fluid. If my fluid gets lower than five percent, there will be no home birth. Instead, I will be induced at the hospital.

I go home. I break into the stash of electrolytes and water we had purchased for the birth. I tell my boss I am not coming back to work and start my maternity leave one week early — one week before my due date — so I can stay home and drink. Water, Gatorade. Gatorade, water. More electrolytes. I eat and drink and flush my sinuses for seven days straight.

One week later, I am still pregnant and back on track for a safe home birth. At the next ultrasound, my fluid level is up. The baby appears to have gained weight. I love her for waiting until I am healthy to drop so that we can do labor better together.

Amy texts, "CHECK YOU OUT!!!!!!!!!!!!!! Nice job! Best patient ever!!!!!!!!!!!!!!!!!" I make a mental note to give her a spirit ribbon when this is over.

Meanwhile, I am a champion. I have beat this sinus infection into oblivion. I am going to have this girl baby like a goddamn warrior and dance victorious under the sun. No, not like a warrior. Like a woman.

Labor begins with 24 hours of boring cramps. Or rather, it feels like the beginning but it's a false start. I lose my mucus plug on Saturday morning, sticky yellow glue that comes out in my underwear. Contractions that night are mild, but strong enough to keep me at home. On Sunday, I walk the length of the house trying to induce contractions, but nothing gets them closer than 10 to 15 minutes apart. After I spend 24 hours pacing the house and killing my second case of Gatorade, two midwives, Dorothy and Annie, make a house call and measure my cervix.

And ... wait for it ... I am four centimeters dilated. Four sad sorry centimeters out of 10. After 24 hours of cramps, I have achieved nothing. I am still so far away from having this baby. I retreat to the bathroom and sob with discouragement. Damn, it sure feels good to cry.

Dorothy thinks that maybe they should sweep my cervical membranes to get the party started. Annie thinks maybe I should drink wine and sleep so that I will be well rested for real labor. "We are going to leave the room now and let you decide," Dorothy says. They retreat. Jacob sits on the bed as my brain splits in two directions. There is the Katy who wants to have her cervix swept. Then there is the Katy who wants to sleep off her frustration of the past 24 hours and push the reset button. Jacob reminds me that it's late, and that I may benefit from a night of sleep.

Because one and a half of us are in favor of rest, rest wins. We say adieu to the midwives. I gulp two melatonin gummies and a small glass of red wine, my first taste of alcohol in almost a year. I draw a warm bath with lavender bubbles, and contractions resume. I have two contractions in the bathtub, then more in the bed after I lie down.

And now the contractions don't stop. It's showtime.

I spend the next few hours under my duvet in an ethereal high from hormones, melatonin and wine. I notice as the contractions come, ride their waves and remain detached. The body's own chemicals are kicking in now, and there's no point in fighting them. I take deep breaths and let them take me.

Sometime in the wee hours, I wake Jacob when the pain becomes intense enough that I don't want to continue laboring alone. I am still lying down, but the contractions are reaching sharp peaks now, piercing through the wine-melatonin-hormone buzz. Jacob calls the midwife on duty and she asks him how far apart my contractions are. Once again, he doesn't know, because he has been sleeping while I labored quietly next to him in bed. He takes my hand and tells me to squeeze his when a contraction hits. I spend most of the next 10 minutes cutting off circulation from his index and middle fingers.

"Okay," I hear Jacob tell her, "she just had three contractions for one to two minutes each." I don't know if that's accurate, but that's what he says.

And with that, two midwives — Marsha and Annie — and Holly are on their way. I hear that news and I feel safe. After months of thoughtful care and conversations, I trust them. They will know what to do. My job is to relax, pay attention to my body and let them take care of the rest.

Holly arrives just as I have risen to my feet to puke in the huge silver mixing bowl Jacob brought from the kitchen, and I am glowing with pride, because I avoided throwing up over the side of the baby's bed, which my fingers are gripping. For bonus points, Jacob won't have to clean up alone this time, because the birth team is coming to our home to help. You are welcome, handsome. Wife of the year.

After that nice big vomit, I get back into bed. I understand now why they write a lot of screaming into childbirth scenes in the movies. Watching a woman cope peacefully with pain never seems to make it in entertainment. There is no drama, no suspense, barely even dialogue. "I couldn't even tell when you were having contractions," Holly will say to me three days postpartum. I am a female cat, quiet in a dark place, letting my body go limp around the rising pain as my uterus does its work. Occasionally, I moan, just to prompt Holly to rub my feet, or signal for Jacob to take my hand and time my contractions. The only evidence of my pain is Jacob's continued loss of circulation from my grip.

What they couldn't see from the outside was that I had found my turtle.

Instead of the animated television shows we humans normally call "cartoons," Enzo's favorite entertainment at age three was BBC's "Planet Earth" documentaries. The episodes are narrated by David Attenborough, whose accent is just about as British as you could hope for. In one episode about the Cape of Good Hope, a clutch of sea turtles hatches. Dozens of tiny turtle babies must rush from their nest in the dry sand to the ocean before they are devoured by yellow billed kites and pine crows who plummet from the sky, or by crabs who snatch them from below the sand's surface.

A small female turtle — the very last hatchling to emerge from this nest — drags herself into the open air with tiny green flippers, blinks the grains of sand from her testudinal eyeballs and flops her vulnerable shell across the beach to the ocean. Against all odds, she avoids death by beak and claw, and reaches the shoreline, where she is drawn into the surf. The danger isn't over: She still has to return to the surface of the water above the pounding waves and draw her first breath before she drowns.

At some point during this second labor, focusing on my breath — and chasing the pain down to its core — became too overwhelming. A healthy microdose of dissociation was necessary. On a poster on the wall of my midwives' office, I had seen a list of tips for active labor. One was visualization. So I had been practicing what I might visualize when contractions hit, and now during labor I went through my inventory. Sunrise on a white-sand beach in Florida? No, suddenly I was terrified of hurricanes. An isolated temple in a lush green forest? No — even as a fantasy, it felt too far away from modern medicine to be safe. My mother's house? No, she would be too nervous at a home birth of her own grandchild. A quiet, dimly lit lounge at a luxury hotel? No, too much effort — even in the fantasy, you would have to be quiet, and wear clean clothes and invisible makeup.

My mind chose a place where I could feel raw, and noisy, and sloppy, and primal.

Baby turtles batting their flippers to escape hungry crows. Baby turtles with sand encrusted in their eyes. Baby turtles gasping for breath in the surf. Baby turtles floating in the deep blue ocean alone on the first day of their lives. Those adorable, tiny, hard-shelled blinking amphibians were my happy place as contractions rose through my body all night and pulled apart my cervix so my daughter could be born. Find your turtle, I told my body. Dig through the sand and find your turtle and walk her to the water and keep her safe. Bring that baby to the surface of the ocean and give her a first breath in this insane, imperfect, glorious, wet world so she can join us.

With each contraction, I mentally cheered my baby on, as she moved millimeters closer to her first breath. With me, and us. On this side of the uterine wall.

Thus went the wee hours of the night, with me summoning my baby sea turtle and the very posh English voice of David Attenborough. I lay on the bed. My gorgeous birth assistant massaged my feet. At one point, I knelt on the floor, head resting on the duvet, while Marsha's hands ran down my naked back, combing out the tension of wound up muscles. After hours of this quiet intimacy, I heard one woman's soft voice tell another, "She says she feels like she is ready to push."

"Katy, let's try another position, okay?" I emerged from my turtle hallucinations and it was now dawn. I was lying facedown on the bed, with my bottom in the air.

My body was switching gears to bear down, like a car going from reverse through neutral and into drive, and for some reason, that raised-butt pose dulled the pain of my contractions. However, the midwives were urging me to lift my chest, so gravity could help the baby descend.

"Noooooooooo!" I growled in protest as the next contraction hit me upright. I clawed my nails against the bedsheets, scratched my mattress like it was the face of a mountain as I tried to avoid the pain of a fall.

Holly found my ear again, just like Lori had done the first time. She was next to me murmuring, "You are almost there, Katy. You are so close. You just have to do one more thing to get this done." Her words knocked me up onto my hands and knees, ready to do the hard work again. I exhaled through gritted teeth and faced the pain again, head-on like a woman.

Damn, I wanted to push. One of the midwives measured me — stealthy like a ninja with her vaginal exam — and told me to wait for a few more contractions. I was still only nine centimeters dilated, but every cell of my body was ready to bear down. After a few more contractions, she told me to go ahead, and I was so thrilled that I exhaled with what felt like all the force of a hurricane. I wanted to flatten my lungs against my diaphragm until there was no space left. I made my breath a jet, multiplying with each contraction to propel the pressure and the pain and the baby onto that bed.

I felt movement.

"Whoa, Katy! That was really fast," Annie said. I could feel fluids coming out, like the amniotic sac had finally popped, and I felt like I was shoving the baby out of my birth canal. But I didn't care. She was head down and her heart was beating and it was time for me to meet her. I set my jaw and gathered up air from every corner of my body and forced my breath down with the next contraction like a rocket. Planet Earth's gravity met me halfway, and let her come.

She was crying. I could still feel the pressure of her shoulders inside my body but I could hear her voice. "Wow. Have you ever seen that before?" one of the midwives said to another. Her head was out. She had taken her first breath. But my work wasn't done. So with the next contraction, I gritted my teeth again, like women do. And my next breath flipped her world inside out.

Now her whole beautiful body was between my legs. Marsha and Annie and Holly helped me roll over onto my back and put her on my belly.

"I did it," I said before anything else. I had made her with my own body, and I had led her out into the surf on my own bed with my own effort and she was here. I sobbed, letting the last seizures of tension go. They passed even more quickly than they had come.

I stared at my baby girl, taking our umbilical cord between my thumb and index finger. It was so wide and went on forever. Ropes of spongy, translucent tissue, the blue thread of blood I could see at its core still flowing from me to her. The midwives would leave it uncut until its pulse stopped.

Suddenly, for the first time in almost 12 hours, my attention wandered. "Where is Enzo?" I said. He had been sleeping in his room all night. His baby sister and I had been on this journey without him. Jacob said he was on the front porch with my dear friend Dee Dee, who had come to care for him. They were waiting for a car to spend the day at her house.

"Go get them," I pleaded. "Bring them in." I needed to hold him, to hold both of these people I had made. Three-year-old Enzo wandered in a minute later, eyes wide, speechless in his little striped red T-shirt, taking in the scene as this coven of women fussed over a wet new human creature who wasn't there the night before. What was that like for him? He may not keep his memories of that day into adulthood, but for a few seconds he saw his mother on the bed naked, a tiny black-haired baby girl on her chest, choking with happiness.

Morning light from the window. The joyful murmurs of strong, kind women as they cleaned up and tended to a new girl in the world. Exhale. Rest.

And then there were four.